COMPLETE GUIDE TO UNDERSTANDING CATARACT SURGERY

Mastering Phacoemulsification, In-Depth Techniques, Recovery Strategies, Expert Insights For Optimal Eye Health And Vision Restoration

KLEIN HOYLE

© [KLEIN HOYLE] [2024]

All rights reserved.

No part of this book may be reproduced, distributed, or transmitted in any form or by any means, including photocopying, recording, or other electronic or mechanical methods, without the publisher's prior written permission, with the exception of brief quotations in critical reviews and certain other noncommercial uses permitted by copyright law.

Disclaimer

The content in this book is based on the author's expertise and comprehension of the topic. The author has no affiliation or link with any corporation, business, or person. This book is meant to give general information and educational material only, and it should not be interpreted as professional medical advice. Always seek the advice of a skilled healthcare expert if you have any queries about medical issues or treatments. The author and publisher expressly disclaim any responsibility resulting directly or indirectly from the use or use of the information included in this book.

Table of Contents

CHAPTER 1 15
Introduction To Cataract Surgery 15
What Is Cataract Surgery? 15
History And Progress Of Cataract Surgery 15
Common Causes And Symptoms Of Cataracts ... 17
Importance Of Cataract Surgery 18

CHAPTER 2 19
Understanding Cataracts 19
Definition And Types Of Cataracts 19
Several Factors May Raise The Chance Of Acquiring Cataracts 20
Impact Of Cataracts On Vision 22
Diagnosis And Evaluation Of Cataract 23

CHAPTER 3 25
Preparing For Surgery 25
Initial Consultation With An Eye Doctor 25
Pre-Operative Tests And Assessments 26
   1. Biometry: 26
   2. Corneal Topography: 27
   3. Dilated Eye Exam: 27

- 4. Visual Acuity exam: 27
- 5. Medical History Review: 27

Medications and Lifestyle Changes Before Surgery 28
- 1. Discontinue Blood-Thinning Medications:..28
- 2. Manage chronic illnesses: 28
- 3. Avoid Eating or Drinking: 28
- 4. Organize transportation: 29

What To Expect On The Day Of Surgery? 29
- 1. Arrival and Registration: 30
- 2. Preparation for Surgery: 30
- 3. Anesthetic: 30
- 4. Surgical Procedure: 30
- 5. Recovery and Discharge: 31

CHAPTER 4 33

Surgical Techniques 33

Overview Of Traditional And Modern Cataract Surgery 33

Phacoemulsification Procedure: Step By Step 34
- 1. Anesthesia: 34
- 2. Incision: 35

3. Capsulorhexis: 35
5. IOL Insertion: 35
6. Wound Closure: 36
7. Postoperative Care: 36
Intraocular Lens (IOL) Options And The Selection Process 36
1. Monofocal IOLs: 36
2. Multifocal IOLs: 37
3. Toric IOLs: 37
4. Accommodating IOLs: 37
Possible Complications And How They Are Managed 38
3. Refractive Errors: 38
CHAPTER 5 41
Anesthesia And Sedation 41
Anesthesia Used In Cataract Surgery 41
Benefits And Risks Of Local Vs. General Anesthesia 42
Sedation Options And Effects 44
Safety Procedures During Anesthesia Administration 45
CHAPTER 6 49

The Surgical Process 49
Operating Room Setup And Sterilization
Procedures 49
Surgical Instruments Used In Cataract Surgery ..51
Incision Techniques And Capsulorhexis............52
Fragmentation And Cataract Removal 54
CHAPTER 7 57
Post-Op Care 57
Immediate Recovery At The Surgical Center 57
Homecare Instructions And Medications..........58
Follow-Up Appointments With The Surgeon 60
Activities And Restrictions For The Healing
Process 61
CHAPTER 8 64
Complications And Risks 64
Common Postoperative Complications............64
Strategies To Prevent Complications................65
Management Of Intraoperative Complications ..67
Long-Term Risks And Implications 68
CHAPTER 9 71
Alternative Treatments..71

An Overview Of Nonsurgical Options For
Cataracts 71
Lifestyle Modifications And Nutritional
Supplements 73
Investigative Therapeutics And Developing
Technologies 75
When Surgery May Not Be Necessary 78
CHAPTER 10 81
Life Following Cataract Surgery 81
Visual Recovery And Adaptation Period 81
Benefits Of Improved Vision Following Surgery 83
   1. Clearer eyesight: 83
   2. Improved Quality of Life: 83
   3. Increased Independence: 84
   4. Reduced Risk of Falls and Accidents: 84
   5. Improved Social Interaction: 84
   6. Better Mental Health: 84
Tips To Maintain Eye Health And Prevent Future
Cataracts 85
   1. Protect Your Eyes from UV Rays: 85
   2. Quit smoking: 86
   3. Consume a Healthy Diet: 86

4. Maintain a Healthy Weight: 86
5. Manage Chronic Conditions: 86
6. Get Regular Eye examinations: 87
Resources For Ongoing Support And Education . 87
1. Support Groups: 87
2. Educational resources: 88
3. Follow-up Care: 88
4. Patient Advocacy Organizations: 88
Conclusion 90
THE END 94

ABOUT THIS BOOK

The "Complete Guide to Understanding Cataract Surgery" is an invaluable reference for anyone navigating the complex terrain of cataract therapy. It digs into every aspect of the surgical process, providing readers with extensive information and assistance.

Chapter 1 introduces readers to the foundations of cataract surgery. This chapter establishes the groundwork for future research, from analyzing the surgical procedure's historical history to describing its relevance in recovering eyesight. It discusses frequent causes and symptoms of cataracts, promoting an educated understanding of the condition's consequences.

Chapter 2 digs further into the complexities of cataracts, explaining their many symptoms and risk factors. This section provides readers with important tools for proactive treatment by explaining the impact of cataracts on vision as well as insights on diagnosis and assessment.

Chapter 3 emphasizes the importance of preparation in achieving a good surgical result. From the first appointment with an eye specialist to pre-operative testing and lifestyle changes, readers are led through the preparation process with clarity and comfort. Patients who understand what to anticipate on the day of surgery may approach the experience with confidence and peace of mind.

Chapter 4 looks into the complexities of surgical methods, contrasting conventional and contemporary approaches. A step-by-step examination of the phacoemulsification method, along with information on intraocular lens alternatives, enables readers to make educated decisions about their treatment plan. By addressing possible difficulties front on, this chapter encourages a proactive approach to post-operative care.

Anesthesia and sedation, discussed in Chapter 5, are critical components of the surgical procedure. Readers acquire a more sophisticated grasp of their choices as the advantages and hazards of different anesthetic techniques are explained. Safety precautions during anesthetic delivery demonstrate the devotion to the patient's well-being and comfort.

The surgical trip begins in Chapter 6 when the operating room setup and sterilization processes are carefully explained. From the complexities of incision procedures to the precise removal of cataracts, readers acquire an understanding of the surgical process's precision and rigor.

Post-operative care, as described in Chapter 7, is critical to achieving optimum recovery and results. From quick recovery in the operating facility to home care instructions and follow-up visits, readers are supported at every stage. Patients who embrace activities and constraints throughout the healing process create an atmosphere favorable to long-term success.

Chapter 8 faces the reality of problems and hazards, recommending solutions for prevention and treatment. This section promotes a proactive approach to post-operative care by encouraging readers to notice warning signals and advocate for their well-being.

Alternative therapies, discussed in Chapter 9, provide a comprehensive approach to cataract care. Readers have access to a varied toolset for tailored treatment, including non-surgical methods, lifestyle changes, and developing technology.

Finally, Chapter 10 depicts life following cataract surgery, highlighting the transformational potential of better eyesight. This section emphasizes the long-term benefits of educated decision-making and proactive self-care by providing practical strategies for preserving eye health and obtaining continuous assistance.

CHAPTER 1

Introduction To Cataract Surgery

What Is Cataract Surgery?

Cataract surgery is a treatment that involves removing a clouded lens from the eye and replacing it with an intraocular lens (IOL). This procedure is usually performed when a cataract affects vision so severely that it interferes with everyday activities and cannot be treated with glasses or contact lenses alone.

The operation is quite simple and is one of the most popular procedures done globally. It is normally done as an outpatient procedure, so you may go home the same day.

History And Progress Of Cataract Surgery

The history of cataract surgery may be traced back thousands of years, with early efforts discovered in ancient civilizations like Egypt and India. However, important improvements in the discipline did not occur until the twentieth century.

One of the most significant advances was the advent of extra capsular cataract extraction (ECCE) in the 1970s, which involved removing the hazy lens while leaving the posterior capsule intact. This procedure enabled the insertion of an IOL, resulting in enhanced visual results.

Surgical procedures evolved throughout time, with the introduction of phacoemulsification in the 1980s, which revolutionized cataract surgery. Phacoemulsification uses ultrasonic waves to break up the cataract, making it simpler to remove via a tiny incision. Because of its effectiveness and safety, this procedure has become the gold standard for cataract surgery.

Common Causes And Symptoms Of Cataracts

Cataracts form when proteins in the lens of the eye clump together, creating cloudiness and opacity. This cloudiness might develop with time, resulting in impaired or poor vision. Common signs of cataracts include:

• Blurred or foggy vision.

• Difficulty seeing at night.

• Sensitive to light and glare.

• Double vision in one eye

• Requires numerous changes in prescription glasses or contact lenses.

Age, heredity, smoking, diabetes, and extended exposure to UV light are all risk factors for cataract formation.

Importance Of Cataract Surgery

Cataract surgery is critical for restoring clear eyesight and increasing the quality of life for those with cataracts. Untreated cataracts may have a major effect on everyday activities such as reading, driving, and doing domestic tasks.

Cataract surgery, which removes the clouded lens and replaces it with an artificial lens, may significantly enhance visual acuity and minimize the need for glasses or contact lenses. Furthermore, early treatment may prevent cataracts from advancing to the point of causing significant vision loss or blindness.

Overall, cataract surgery is a safe and effective operation that provides life-changing advantages to patients with cataracts.

CHAPTER 2

Understanding Cataracts

Definition And Types Of Cataracts

Cataracts are a frequent eye ailment that affects the lens, which is a transparent component inside the eye. They arise when proteins in the lens start to clump together, resulting in cloudiness or opacity. This cloudiness might develop over time, resulting in visual impairment.

Cataracts are classified into various categories, each with distinct characteristics:

1. Age-related cataracts are the most prevalent kind of cataract and arise naturally as people age. As we age, the proteins in our lenses become less flexible and more prone to clumping together, resulting in cataracts.

2. Congenital cataracts occur in newborns or children and might be present from birth or develop soon after. They may be caused by genetics, pregnancy-related illnesses, or other medical issues.

3. Secondary cataracts may occur as a consequence of diabetes, exposure to certain drugs, such as steroids, or ocular damage.

4. Traumatic cataracts are caused by physical damage to the eye, such as blunt force trauma or piercing injuries.

Understanding the kind of cataract a person has is critical for identifying the best treatment technique.

Risk Factors for Developing Cataracts:

Several Factors May Raise The Chance Of Acquiring Cataracts

1. Cataracts are more likely to form as individuals become older, with the majority of instances happening in those over 60.

2. Family History: Genetics may influence the development of cataracts. If you have a family history of cataracts, you may be at a greater risk.

3. UV Radiation: Prolonged exposure to ultraviolet (UV) radiation from the sun increases the risk of cataracts. Wearing UV-protective eyewear may assist in lessening this risk.

4. Smoking and heavy alcohol intake have been related to a higher incidence of cataracts.

5. Medical Conditions: Diabetes, hypertension, and obesity may all raise the chance of getting cataracts.

6. drugs: Certain drugs, including corticosteroids and statins, have been linked to an increased risk of cataracts.

7. Eye Trauma: Previous eye injuries or operations enhance the likelihood of acquiring cataracts later in life.

Understanding these risk factors may help people make efforts to lower their chances of acquiring cataracts and keep their eyes healthy.

Impact Of Cataracts On Vision

Cataracts may significantly impair eyesight, depending on their severity and placement inside the lens. Cataracts often affect eyesight in the following ways:

1. Cloudy Vision: Cataracts may produce impaired or cloudy vision, making it difficult to see properly.

2. Cataracts may cause an increase in sensitivity to bright lights or glare, making it difficult to remain in well-lit areas.

3. Difficulty Seeing at Night: Cataracts may make it difficult to see properly in low-light situations, such as at night or in poorly lit rooms.

4. Changes in Color Vision: Some persons with cataracts may notice that colors seem faded or yellowed.

5. Double Vision: Cataracts may sometimes produce double vision or visual ghosting, making it difficult to concentrate on things.

Understanding how cataracts impair vision may help people identify symptoms and seek suitable treatment.

Diagnosis And Evaluation Of Cataract

An ophthalmologist or optometrist often performs a full eye examination to diagnose cataracts. During the examination, the eye doctor will run numerous tests to check the eye's health and the amount of the cataract, such as:

1. The Visual Acuity Test uses an eye chart to determine how well you can see at different distances.

2. Slit-lamp Examination: The doctor will use a special microscope known as a slit lamp to check the

eye's structures, especially the lens, for evidence of cataracts.

3. Retinal Examination: The doctor may dilate your pupils and check the back of your eye, including the retina, to detect any other eye diseases.

4. Tonometry: This test monitors pressure within the eye and is used to screen for glaucoma, which may coexist with cataracts.

5. Visual Field exam: This exam evaluates your peripheral vision and may reveal visual field loss caused by cataracts.

Once a cataract is discovered, the eye doctor will discuss treatment options depending on the severity of the cataract and the patient's visual requirements.

CHAPTER 3

Preparing For Surgery

Initial Consultation With An Eye Doctor

Your route to cataract surgery usually starts with an initial consultation with an eye specialist. This is an important phase in which you will discuss your symptoms, medical history, and any questions you may have concerning the operation. The eye specialist will do a thorough eye examination to establish the severity of your cataracts and if surgery is required.

During the appointment, the doctor will discuss the many kinds of intraocular lenses (IOLs) available and assist you in selecting the best choice depending on your lifestyle and visual requirements. They will answer any questions or concerns you have concerning the operation, anesthesia, recuperation, and any dangers.

This session allows you to express your expectations and wishes about the result of the procedure. The doctor will give you reasonable expectations for the improvements in your eyesight following the treatment.

Following the consultation, you will have a greater grasp of the whole process and be more prepared for what comes next.

Pre-Operative Tests And Assessments

Before having cataract surgery, you will need to go through numerous pre-operative tests and evaluations to determine that you are a good candidate for the treatment and to obtain important information to guide the surgical process.

These tests may include:

1. **Biometry:** This test assesses the size and shape of your eye to calculate the power of the intraocular lens (IOL) that will be inserted after surgery.

2. Corneal Topography: This test measures the curvature of your cornea, which is critical for determining the right IOL power and analyzing the health of your cornea.

3. Dilated Eye Exam: Eye drops will dilate your pupils, allowing the doctor to completely examine the lens and retina in the rear of your eye.

4. Visual Acuity exam: This common eye chart exam determines how well you can see at different distances, which helps in determining the severity of your cataract-related visual impairment.

5. Medical History Review: The doctor will examine your medical history to see if there are any underlying health concerns or drugs that might impact the operation or anesthesia.

These tests are critical for tailoring the surgery approach to your specific requirements and achieving the best possible results.

Medications and Lifestyle Changes Before Surgery

In the days or weeks before your cataract surgery, your doctor may prescribe specific drugs or lifestyle changes to improve your health and lower the chance of problems during and after the operation.

You could be urged to:

1. **Discontinue Blood-Thinning Medications:** If you're taking aspirin or warfarin, your doctor may advise you to stop or reduce your dose before surgery to reduce the chance of bleeding during the operation.

2. **Manage chronic illnesses:** If you have illnesses such as diabetes or high blood pressure, it is critical to keep them under control before surgery to aid healing and decrease the chance of complications.

3. **Avoid Eating or Drinking:** Because anesthetic is often used during the process, you will usually be told to

refrain from eating or drinking for many hours before the surgery.

4. **Organize transportation:** Because you will most likely be unable to drive immediately after surgery due to the effects of anesthetic and potential blurriness in your vision, you must organize transportation to and from the medical facility.

Following this advice and making the appropriate changes to your lifestyle and medicines can help guarantee a smoother surgery experience and increase the probability of a positive result.

What To Expect On The Day Of Surgery?

The day of your cataract surgery will most likely be filled with anticipation and nervousness, but knowing what to anticipate may help ease some of the worry and make the procedure seem more manageable.

Here's a broad description of what usually occurs on the day before surgery:

1. Arrival and Registration: You will arrive at the surgery facility and fill out any required paperwork or registration forms. You may also meet with the surgical team to review the operation and discuss any last-minute questions or concerns.

2. Preparation for Surgery: Before the operation starts, you will be prepared, which may involve changing into a surgical gown and having your vital signs taken. You will also be given eye medications to dilate your pupils and numb the eye.

3. Anesthetic: Most cataract procedures are conducted with local anesthetic, which means you will be awake but your eye will be numbed to avoid pain. You may be given a sedative to help you relax throughout the treatment.

4. Surgical Procedure: After you've been prepped and the anesthetic has taken effect, the surgeon will begin the cataract removal procedure. Typically, a tiny incision is made in the eye, and the clouded lens is broken up with ultrasound energy before being removed. The surgeon will next implant a clear artificial lens to replace the natural one.

5. Recovery and Discharge: Following the procedure, you will spend some time in a recovery area where the surgical team will check your vital signs and make sure you are comfortable. When you are awake and stable, you will be released with post-operative instructions and any required medicines.

Overall, cataract surgery is a short and simple treatment with a high success rate and little pain. Knowing what to anticipate on the day of surgery allows you to approach the procedure with confidence and concentrate on the benefits it will bring to your eyesight and quality of life.

CHAPTER 4
Surgical Techniques

Overview Of Traditional And Modern Cataract Surgery

Cataract surgery has advanced dramatically from ancient procedures to current ones, resulting in better patient outcomes and recuperation periods. Traditional cataract surgery involves creating a bigger incision in the eye, physically removing the hazy lens, and replacing it with an intraocular lens. While successful, this method often necessitates longer downtime and has a greater risk of problems such as astigmatism and induced astigmatism.

In contrast, current cataract surgery is usually performed using a procedure known as phacoemulsification. This minimally invasive method includes making a small incision in the cornea and inserting an ultrasonic probe to break up the clouded lens into small pieces. These pieces are then suctioned out of the eye, making way for the implantation of a foldable IOL via the same tiny incision. Phacoemulsification has many benefits over typical surgery, including speedier recovery, a lower risk of complications, and better visual results.

Phacoemulsification Procedure: Step By Step

Phacoemulsification is the most often utilized procedure in contemporary cataract surgery owing to its accuracy and efficacy. Here's a step-by-step explanation of how the operation is normally carried out:

1. Anesthesia: Before surgery, the eye is numbed with either topical anesthesia (eye drops) or a local anesthetic injection around the eye. This guarantees the patient's comfort throughout the process.

2. **Incision:** A tiny incision, usually less than 3 millimeters wide, is created in the cornea. This incision allows surgical tools to enter the inside of the eye.

3. **Capsulorhexis:** A circular opening is made in the front region of the lens capsule using a specific instrument known as a cystotome or capsulorhexis forceps. This hole enables the surgeon to reach and remove the clouded lens.

4. Phacoemulsification involves inserting an ultrasonic probe via an incision into the eye. The probe uses high-frequency sound waves to break up the hazy lens into small pieces, which are subsequently suctioned out of the eye.

5. **IOL Insertion:** Once the cataract has been completely removed, an artificial intraocular lens (IOL) is put via the same tiny incision. The IOL unfolds within the eye and is positioned to replace the natural lens's focusing ability.

6. Wound Closure: In most situations, the little incision heals on its own without the need for sutures. The eye is allowed to recover naturally, lowering postoperative pain and the danger of infection.

7. Postoperative Care: Following surgery, the patient may get eye drops or drugs to avoid infection and irritation. Follow-up sessions are arranged to evaluate healing progress and check visual acuity.

Intraocular Lens (IOL) Options And The Selection Process

Choosing the appropriate intraocular lens (IOL) is an important step in cataract surgery since it directly affects the patient's visual result and quality of life. There are various varieties of IOLs available, each with its characteristics and benefits:

1. Monofocal IOLs: These lenses provide clear vision at a single focal distance, usually distant or near vision. Patients who choose mono-focal IOLs may still need glasses for tasks like reading or driving, depending on the focal point of the lens.

2. Multifocal IOLs: Multifocal lenses improve vision at many distances, decreasing the need for glasses or contact lenses after surgery. These lenses may give good vision for both nearby and distant objects, improving overall visual acuity and convenience.

3. Toric IOLs: These lenses are intended to correct astigmatism, a common refractive problem that may result in blurry or distorted vision. Toric IOLs may increase visual clarity and minimize the need for glasses by treating cataracts and astigmatism at the same time.

4. Accommodating IOLs: These lenses are intended to mirror the natural focusing capacity of the eye's crystalline lens, allowing for smooth transitions between distances without the need for reading glasses. For individuals with presbyopia, these lenses improve depth of focus and visual flexibility.

Possible Complications And How They Are Managed

While cataract surgery is typically safe and successful, like with any surgical operation, there is some risk of problems. Common problems may include:

1. Intraoperative complications may arise during surgery, such as injury to the eye's surrounding tissues or partial cataract removal. Intraoperative problems are often addressed immediately by the surgeon to minimize their influence on the ultimate visual result.

2. Patients may encounter postoperative problems such as infection, irritation, or corneal edema. These problems are routinely treated with antibiotics or anti-inflammatory eye medicines, as well as constant monitoring by the surgical team.

3. **Refractive Errors:** Some individuals may develop residual refractive errors after cataract surgery, including nearsightedness, farsightedness, or

astigmatism. These defects may often be repaired with glasses, contact lenses, or other surgical treatments such as laser vision correction.

4. Secondary Cataracts: Some individuals may develop a disease known as posterior capsule opacification (PCO) months or years after cataract surgery, which causes their eyesight to become clouded again. PCO may be treated with a short and painless laser operation called YAG capsulotomy, which eliminates the cloudiness and restores clear vision.

Patients may make educated treatment choices and have confidence in the safety and efficacy of cataract surgery if they understand the possible problems and how they are addressed. Close communication with the surgical team, as well as adherence to postoperative care recommendations, are critical for improving results and reducing the risk of complications.

CHAPTER 5

Anesthesia And Sedation

Anesthesia Used In Cataract Surgery

Cataract surgery normally uses two forms of anesthesia: local and general. A local anesthetic numbs the eye region, but general anesthesia causes unconsciousness for the length of the treatment.

Local anesthetic is often provided by eye drops or injections around the eye. These drugs inhibit the sense of pain in the eye and surrounding tissues, enabling the patient to stay awake and attentive during the procedure. Many people choose local anesthetic because it removes the hazards of general anesthesia and allows for a quicker recovery.

General anesthesia, on the other hand, is provided intravenously or by inhalation, allowing the patient to lose consciousness and experience no discomfort throughout the procedure. While general anesthesia may be required for individuals who cannot tolerate local anesthetics or have certain medical conditions, it is associated with a greater risk of complications such as respiratory issues and allergic responses.

Benefits And Risks Of Local Vs. General Anesthesia

Local anesthetic provides various advantages for cataract surgery patients. It provides for a faster recovery period, lowers the risk of problems associated with general anesthesia, and allows patients to speak with the surgical team during the process. Furthermore, local anesthesia is often selected for individuals with underlying medical issues or who are at a greater risk of complications from general anesthesia.

However, there are potential hazards connected with local anesthesia. While uncommon, possible risks include eye irritation, allergic responses to anesthetic drugs, and increased intraocular pressure. Patients with specific medical disorders, such as acute anxiety or claustrophobia, may struggle to stay quiet and motionless throughout the procedure under local anesthetic.

General anesthesia, on the other hand, guarantees that the patient is entirely asleep and painless during the procedure. This may be useful for individuals who are nervous about the surgery or have trouble sitting still for a lengthy amount of time. Furthermore, general anesthesia enables the surgical team to execute more complicated surgeries or handle many eye diseases at once.

However, general anesthesia entails a larger risk of problems than local anesthetic. Breathing issues, allergic reactions, and postoperative nausea and vomiting are all potential dangers. Patients with specific medical disorders, such as heart or lung illness, may be more likely to have complications from general anesthesia.

Sedation Options And Effects

In addition to anesthetic, individuals undergoing cataract surgery may be given sedation to help them relax and feel more at ease throughout the treatment. Sedation levels may vary from light to severe, depending on the patient's requirements and preferences.

Intravenous (IV) sedation is a typical sedation method in which drugs are administered via a vein to promote relaxation and sleepiness. IV sedation enables patients to be aware and responsive throughout surgery while feeling calm and comfortable. This sort of sedation is sometimes used for individuals who are nervous about the treatment or have difficulties staying still for a lengthy amount of time.

Another sedation option is oral sedation, which is taking medicine orally to produce calm and lessen anxiety before the operation. Oral sedation is often gentler than IV sedation and may be appropriate for people with mild to moderate anxiety or those who do not want to take medicine via IV.

Regardless of the sedation method selected, patients should discuss their preferences and medical history with their physician before the treatment. This enables the surgical team to adjust the anesthetic and sedation strategy to the patient's specific requirements, ensuring a safe and pleasant surgical procedure.

Safety Procedures During Anesthesia Administration

Several precautions are taken during cataract surgery to ensure that anesthesia and sedation are administered safely. Before the surgery, the surgical team will examine the patient's medical history, including any allergies or underlying health concerns, to select the best anesthetic and sedative alternatives.

During the operation, the anesthesia provider will continuously monitor the patient's vital signs, such as heart rate, blood pressure, and oxygen levels, to ensure that they stay stable and within acceptable limits. Furthermore, the surgical team will be ready to respond rapidly to any bad reactions or problems that may occur during the treatment.

Before providing anesthesia, the anesthesia professional will describe the process and answer any questions or concerns the patient may have. To limit the risk of problems, patients must strictly adhere to their surgeon's preoperative instructions, which may include fasting before surgery.

Following surgery, patients will be constantly observed throughout the recovery period to ensure that they are awake and attentive and that their vital signs are stable. Any postoperative pain or discomfort will be controlled with appropriate drugs, and patients will be given follow-up care instructions as well as any activity limitations that may be required.

Overall, the patient's safety and comfort are top priorities during cataract surgery, and the surgical team will take every measure to achieve a satisfactory result. Complications may be avoided and the risk of adverse events decreased by carefully choosing the right anesthetic and sedative alternatives and continuously monitoring the patient during the treatment.

CHAPTER 6

The Surgical Process

Operating Room Setup And Sterilization Procedures

The operating room (OR) setting is critical for maintaining a safe and sanitary environment during cataract surgery. Before the procedure, the OR team thoroughly prepares the area to reduce the risk of infection and problems.

First, the OR is carefully cleansed and disinfected to eliminate any possible sources of infection. All surfaces, including the operation table, equipment, and surrounding surroundings, are sterilized with medical-grade disinfectants.

Sterilization processes are then carried out to guarantee that all tools and equipment used during surgery are free of hazardous bacteria.

This entails utilizing autoclaves or other sterilization procedures to heat and destroy any bacteria, viruses, or fungus on the equipment.

Once the OR is ready, the surgical team puts on sterile gowns, gloves, masks, and helmets to avoid contamination throughout the surgery. Proper hand cleanliness is also done to reduce the possibility of infections entering the surgical site.

In addition to maintaining a clean environment, the OR setup entails situating the patient comfortably on the operating table and providing appropriate lighting and ventilation for the surgical team to conduct the surgery successfully.

Overall, thorough attention to detail in OR setup and sterilization protocols is critical for lowering infection risk and assuring excellent results in cataract surgery.

Surgical Instruments Used In Cataract Surgery

Cataract surgery necessitates the use of sophisticated devices intended to securely and accurately remove the clouded lens from the eye and implant a clean prosthetic lens. These devices play an important role in aiding several aspects of the surgical process.

The phacoemulsification handpiece is a key tool in cataract surgery because it uses ultrasonic energy to break up the cataract into small pieces that can be readily aspirated from the eye. This portable instrument enables the surgeon to move softly within the eye while minimizing harm to surrounding tissues.

Another useful tool is the intraocular lens (IOL) injector, which is used to implant the artificial lens into the eye after the cataract has been removed. The injector inserts the folded IOL via a tiny incision and unfolds it into the proper place inside the eye.

Microsurgical equipment such as forceps, scissors, and manipulators are also used during cataract surgery to help with incisions, capsulorhexis (an opening in the lens capsule), and intraocular tissue manipulation.

Furthermore, specialized equipment like viscoelastic devices and irrigation/aspiration probes are utilized to keep intraocular pressure stable and irrigate the surgical region during the surgery.

The selection and careful usage of surgical equipment are crucial for attaining the best results in cataract surgery. Surgeons and their staff go through intensive training to master the use of this equipment and guarantee that each surgery is safe and successful.

Incision Techniques And Capsulorhexis

Precise incisions and capsulorhexis are critical components of cataract surgery because they enable the surgeon to access and securely remove the cataractous lens from the eye.

Several approaches are used to make incisions and capsulorhexis during the treatment.

Small, self-sealing incisions are often created on the cornea's perimeter to reduce induced astigmatism and facilitate speedier healing. These incisions are precisely sized and placed to provide access to the lens while preserving the structural integrity of the eye.

Capsulorhexis, or the formation of a circular hole in the lens capsule, is used to access and remove the cataract. This process requires precision and control to ensure that the aperture is the proper size and located inside the capsular bag.

Capsulorhexis may be achieved in a variety of ways, including manual ripping with forceps, mechanical capsulorhexis devices, and femtosecond laser technologies. Each procedure has benefits and disadvantages, and the technique used is determined by criteria such as surgeon preference, patient anatomy, and technological availability.

Regardless of the approach utilized, capsulorhexis is an important step in cataract surgery because it creates a clean channel for accessing and removing the cataractous lens and enables for precise implantation of the intraocular lens (IOL) implant.

Surgeons get significant training and experience to perfect incision methods and capsulorhexis, ensuring that each stage of the surgical operation is executed with precision and care to obtain the best possible results for the patient.

Fragmentation And Cataract Removal

The primary goals of cataract surgery are to fragment and remove the cataractous lens, restoring clarity and vision to the patient's eye. Several strategies and technologies are used to attain this aim safely and efficiently.

Phacoemulsification is the most popular method for fragmenting and eliminating cataracts during surgery.

This procedure uses ultrasonic energy to break up the cataract into little fragments that can be aspirated from the eye using suction.

The phacoemulsification handpiece, which includes a tiny ultrasonic probe, is put into the eye via a small incision, enabling the surgeon to emulsify the cataract and remove the pieces while minimizing harm to the surrounding tissues.

In certain circumstances, sophisticated procedures like femtosecond laser-assisted cataract surgery may be used to fragment the cataract before phacoemulsification. This method employs laser radiation to accurately break the cataract into tiny pieces, making removal more precise and efficient.

Following the fragmentation and removal of the cataract from the eye, an artificial intraocular lens (IOL) is implanted to replace the natural lens and restore vision.

The IOL is gently put into the capsular bag or another area inside the eye, where it is fixed in place.

Throughout the fragmentation and removal process, the surgical team checks the eye's intraocular pressure, fluid balance, and general health to guarantee the procedure's safety and success. To get the best results and restore the patient's eyesight, painstaking attention to detail and modern surgical procedures are used.

CHAPTER 7

Post-Op Care

Immediate Recovery At The Surgical Center

The first recuperation time after cataract surgery is critical for a seamless transition from the operating room to the postoperative period. Typically, patients are carefully followed in a dedicated recovery room inside the operating facility. Medical personnel monitor vital signs, evaluate for any urgent difficulties, and provide drugs or treatments to ensure comfort and safety.

During this period, patients may suffer typical post-operative symptoms like slight pain, tears, or blurred vision. These symptoms are typically transitory and normal as the eyes adapt to the surgical modifications. However, if there is extreme pain, abrupt vision loss, or any other troubling symptoms, it is critical to inform medical personnel right once for urgent diagnosis and treatment.

The length of the recovery time at the surgical center will vary based on individual circumstances such as the kind of anesthetic used, any pre-existing medical issues, and the complexity of the surgery. When the patient is pronounced stable and ready for release, they will be given specific instructions for home care and follow-up visits.

Homecare Instructions And Medications

Following release from the surgery facility, patients are given detailed home care instructions to enhance recovery and reduce the chance of problems. These instructions usually contain suggestions for eye cleanliness, medication management, and activity limitations during the early healing period.

One of the most important components of home care following cataract surgery is the careful administration of prescription eye drops. These drops are essential in avoiding infection, decreasing inflammation, and encouraging recovery. Patients are trained on the frequency and duration of each kind of eye drop, as well as the precise instillation method, to ensure maximum efficacy.

In addition to eye drops, patients may be offered oral drugs such as antibiotics or pain relievers, depending on their specific requirements. It is critical to stick to the recommended medication regimen and any particular instructions supplied by the surgeon to promote the healing process and manage any post-operative pain.

Along with medication treatment, patients should maintain proper eye care to limit the risk of infection and other problems. This may include gently washing the eyelids and avoiding activities that might bring dirt or debris into the eyes during the first healing process.

Follow-Up Appointments With The Surgeon

Follow-up meetings with the surgeon are an essential component of post-operative care after cataract surgery. These consultations enable the surgeon to check on the healing process, measure visual acuity, and address any concerns or difficulties that may occur throughout the recovery time.

Typically, the initial follow-up visit is arranged between a few days and a week following surgery. During this appointment, the surgeon will inspect the eyes, remove any leftover sutures as needed, and assess the overall effectiveness of the surgery. Patients may be subjected to further tests or imaging investigations to evaluate the intraocular lens location and guarantee adequate alignment for the best visual results.

Follow-up sessions are arranged regularly to assess long-term results and manage any late-onset problems, such as posterior capsule opacification or refractive error. The frequency of these checkups may vary based on individual circumstances and the surgeon's recommendations.

Activities And Restrictions For The Healing Process

During the early healing period after cataract surgery, patients are encouraged to follow particular activities and limits to achieve optimum results and reduce the risk of problems. While it is important to follow the particular directions supplied by the surgeon, here are some basic guidelines:

• Avoid rubbing or touching the eyes as it might lead to infection or dislodgement of the intraocular lens. Patients should avoid rubbing their eyes and use care while administering eye drops or doing anything near their eyes.

- Avoid strenuous activities such as heavy lifting, bending, and exercising during the early healing period to prevent eye strain or pressure. Patients should also avoid engaging in activities that may expose their eyes to dust, dirt, or other pollutants.

- Protect eyes from bright light, since it might create pain and sensitivity throughout the healing process. Wearing sunglasses or protective eyewear outside and limiting exposure to bright lights inside might help relieve these symptoms.

- Follow Driving Restrictions: Patients may be recommended to avoid driving for a time after cataract surgery, particularly if there are lingering visual abnormalities or if both eyes were operated on simultaneously. To ensure safety and the best visual recovery, adhere to the surgeon's instructions for driving limitations.

- Regular follow-up sessions with the surgeon are essential for evaluating healing progress and resolving any problems. Patients should adhere to the suggested follow-up visit schedule and quickly notify the medical team of any changes in symptoms or visual acuity.

Patients who follow these instructions and adhere to the suggested post-operative care routine may assist in ensuring a smooth recovery and the best potential visual results after cataract surgery.

CHAPTER 8
Complications And Risks

Common Postoperative Complications

Following cataract surgery, individuals may encounter a few typical post-operative problems, which are usually minor and easily curable. Inflammation is one kind of problem that may cause redness, discomfort, and impaired vision. This inflammation usually fades with anti-inflammatory eye drops provided by the surgeon. Another possible risk is a rise in eye pressure, known as ocular hypertension, which might result from the body's reaction to the procedure. This is often treated with eye drops or other drugs.

Another risk is posterior capsule opacification (PCO), in which the capsule behind the intraocular lens becomes hazy, causing visual issues comparable to those that existed before to surgery.

However, this is readily remedied with a laser operation known as YAG laser capsulotomy, which makes a hole in the clouded capsule and restores clear vision. Furthermore, some individuals may develop acute corneal swelling or edema, which may cause impaired vision and pain but often resolves on its own or with the use of prescription eye drops.

Infection, hemorrhage, retinal detachment, and vision loss are all rare consequences, occurring in just a tiny proportion of patients. To reduce the risk of problems, patients must carefully follow their surgeon's instructions following surgery and report any unexpected symptoms as soon as they appear.

Strategies To Prevent Complications

To reduce the risk of problems after cataract surgery, numerous techniques may be used. Preoperative evaluation is critical because it lets the surgeon detect any possible risk factors, such as pre-existing eye disorders or systemic illnesses, that might increase the possibility of complications. Proper patient education is also necessary, as patients must understand the significance of following post-operative recommendations for medication usage, eye protection, and activity limitations.

Keeping the operating room clean and using modern procedures like phacoemulsification may help lower the risk of infection and other intraoperative problems. Furthermore, employing high-quality intraocular lenses and carefully determining the right lens power for each patient helps reduce the risk of post-operative refractive errors and other visual problems.

Patients must be closely monitored after surgery, and any problems must be addressed as soon as possible. Patients should be encouraged to attend all follow-up sessions and report any unexpected symptoms, such as extreme pain, abrupt visual changes, or evidence of infection, as soon as possible. By using these techniques, the occurrence of problems may be considerably minimized, resulting in improved results for cataract surgery patients.

Management Of Intraoperative Complications

Although cataract surgery is typically safe, intraoperative problems can arise. One such consequence is a posterior capsule tear, which occurs when the capsule enclosing the cataract is injured during the procedure. This might result in the loss of vitreous fluid, necessitating further surgical procedures, such as anterior vitrectomy, to remove the vitreous and avoid consequences such as retinal detachment.

Another intraoperative complication is a nucleus drop, which occurs when the cataract nucleus slips into the back of the eye during the procedure. This may be difficult to handle, however, approaches like viscoelastic injection or the use of specialist devices may be necessary to securely recover the nucleus.

Other potential intraoperative problems include iris trauma, zonular dehiscence, and Descemet's membrane separation, all of which need careful treatment to reduce the risk of future eye injury and provide the best possible visual results for the patient. Surgeons must be prepared to manage these issues quickly and efficiently during surgery to limit the risk of long-term complications and vision loss.

Long-Term Risks And Implications

While cataract surgery is very effective in improving eyesight and quality of life for the majority of people, there are some long-term concerns to be aware of. One such concern is the development of posterior capsule opacification (PCO), as previously stated, which may occur months or even years following surgery. Although PCO is readily treated with simple laser surgery, it may still impair visual function and may need extensive follow-up treatment.

Another long-term danger is the advancement of underlying eye disorders such as age-related macular degeneration (AMD) or glaucoma, which may continue to impair vision even after successful cataract surgery. Patients with these diseases may need regular monitoring and therapy to keep their eyesight stable and avoid future deterioration.

Furthermore, some patients may be dissatisfied with their visual results after cataract surgery, such as residual refractive errors or visual disturbances like halos or glare, particularly in low-light circumstances. These difficulties are often resolved using glasses or contact lenses; but, in rare circumstances, further surgical operations may be required to obtain the requisite visual acuity.

Overall, although cataract surgery is seen to be safe and successful, patients should be informed of the possible long-term dangers and schedule frequent eye examinations to check their vision and overall eye health.

CHAPTER 9

Alternative Treatments

An Overview Of Nonsurgical Options For Cataracts

Cataracts are often connected with age and develop when the normal lens of the eye gets clouded. While surgery is the most frequent and successful therapy for cataracts, there are several non-surgical alternatives, particularly in the early stages of the disease.

One of the easiest non-surgical treatments is to treat cataract symptoms using prescription glasses or contact lenses. These corrective lenses may assist enhance vision by adjusting for cataract-related cloudiness. However, it should be noted that this is simply a temporary remedy and does not address the underlying cause of the cataract.

Prescription eye drops are another nonsurgical treatment option for cataracts. These drops usually include antioxidants or other chemicals that are thought to decrease the formation of cataracts or alleviate their symptoms. While research into the efficacy of these eye drops is continuing, certain trials have shown encouraging outcomes in specific circumstances.

In addition to prescription eye drops, some individuals may benefit from taking over-the-counter supplements including vitamins C and E, as well as minerals such as selenium and zinc. These nutrients are known to have antioxidant qualities, which might help protect the eyes from cataract-related damage. However, before beginning any new supplement program, contact with a healthcare practitioner, since they may interfere with other prescriptions or have negative effects.

Lifestyle adjustments like as stopping smoking, eating a nutritious diet, and wearing UV-blocking eyewear may help prevent the growth of cataracts and alleviate their symptoms. While these approaches may not remove the need for surgery in the long term, they may nevertheless be useful components of a complete cataract management strategy.

Lifestyle Modifications And Nutritional Supplements

Making lifestyle modifications and including dietary supplements in your daily routine may help manage cataracts and perhaps halt their advancement.

First and foremost, eating a nutritious diet rich in fruits, vegetables, and whole grains may supply important nutrients for eye health. Antioxidant-rich foods, such as leafy greens, citrus fruits, and berries, may help protect the eyes from free radical damage and oxidative stress, both of which are thought to contribute to cataract formation.

In addition to a balanced diet, several dietary supplements may be useful to those who have cataracts. Antioxidant vitamins including vitamin C, vitamin E, and beta-carotene have been investigated for their ability to lower the risk of cataract development or decrease the advancement of existing cataracts. Minerals such as selenium and zinc may also help to promote general eye health.

However, although dietary supplements might help you live a healthier lifestyle, they are not a replacement for medical care. Before beginning a new supplement regimen, contact with a healthcare expert to confirm that it is safe and suitable for your specific requirements.

In addition to nutritional issues, several lifestyle choices may influence eye health and cataract advancement. For example, smoking has been related to an increased risk of cataract formation and progression, thus quitting may be a significant step in managing the disease. Furthermore, shielding your eyes from UV radiation by wearing sunglasses outside and avoiding prolonged sun exposure might help prevent future eye damage.

By adopting these lifestyle modifications and nutritional supplements into your daily routine, you may take proactive actions to improve eye health and perhaps halt the growth of cataracts. However, keep in mind that these steps should be taken in combination with routine eye examinations and medical therapy as prescribed by your healthcare professional.

Investigative Therapeutics And Developing Technologies

While cataract surgery is still the gold standard for treating cataracts, researchers are always looking into novel medicines and technology that might provide alternative or complementary methods to control the problem.

One area of active study is the development of pharmacological medicines capable of being administered directly to the eye and targeting the underlying processes of cataract formation. These treatments might include antioxidants, anti-inflammatory medicines, or chemicals that prevent the formation of eye proteins linked to cataracts. By targeting particular pathways involved in cataract formation, these medicines hope to halt the advancement of the disorder or perhaps prevent cataracts from developing in the first place.

In addition to pharmaceutical therapies, researchers are looking at the possibility of new technologies like laser therapy and ultrasound therapy to cure cataracts. Laser-assisted cataract surgery, for example, employs a femtosecond laser to make precise incisions in the eye and fracture the hazy lens, making it simpler to remove. Similarly, ultrasonic treatment uses high-frequency sound waves to emulsify and remove the lens from the eye.

These developing technologies have the potential to improve the precision and efficiency of cataract surgery, resulting in fewer risks and quicker recovery for patients. However, further study is required to properly evaluate their safety and efficacy when compared to standard cataract surgery.

Overall, although cataract surgery is still the most effective therapy for cataracts, continuous research into experimental medicines and developing technology provide promise for alternate or complementary ways to control the disease. Individuals with cataracts may keep updated about these discoveries and collaborate closely with healthcare experts to investigate all available choices for preserving vision and maintaining general eye health.

When Surgery May Not Be Necessary

Cataract surgery is widely regarded as both safe and successful in repairing visual impairment caused by cataracts. However, in other cases, surgery may not be indicated or may need to be postponed.

Surgery may not be advised if the cataract has no major effect on vision or causes considerable discomfort. In some circumstances, the dangers of surgery may exceed the benefits, and healthcare experts may advise patients to monitor the cataract and consider surgery only if their vision deteriorates or symptoms worsen.

Similarly, people with certain medical or ocular issues may not be suitable candidates for cataract surgery. Uncontrolled diabetes, severe glaucoma, or extensive macular degeneration may all raise the risks of surgery and reduce the probability of success. In some circumstances, healthcare experts may suggest different therapies or management measures for visual impairment.

Individuals who are unable to have surgery because of other health issues or personal preferences can consider non-surgical methods for cataract management, such as prescription glasses, contact lenses, or lifestyle modifications. While these methods may not completely remove the cataract, they may assist improve vision and quality of life for certain people with mild to moderate cataracts.

Finally, the choice to have cataract surgery should be taken in collaboration with a healthcare professional, who can evaluate specific circumstances and explain the possible risks and advantages of the operation. Individuals suffering from cataracts may make educated choices regarding their eye care and vision therapy by carefully assessing these considerations and researching all available solutions.

CHAPTER 10

Life Following Cataract Surgery

Visual Recovery And Adaptation Period

Patients who have had cataract surgery often have a period of visual recovery and adaptation. This phase differs from one to person, but knowing what to anticipate will help alleviate any fears.

Patients often report blurriness or haziness in their vision immediately after surgery. This is common while the eye recovers after the operation. Vision may take a few days to completely settle, and in some circumstances, many weeks to get ideal results.

During the healing time, patients should carefully follow their doctor's recommendations. This may include using prescription eye drops, wearing a protective eye shield at night, and avoiding activities that might strain the eyes, such as heavy lifting or rubbing them.

As the eye recovers, individuals' eyesight may improve. Colors may look more bright, while objects may appear sharper and more defined. Some people may also notice an improvement in their night vision or low-light circumstances.

It is crucial to realize that, although cataract surgery may considerably improve eyesight, it may not be flawless. Some people may still need glasses or contact lenses for certain tasks like reading or driving. Your doctor will review your visual demands and provide suggestions based on your unique situation.

During the adaptation phase, it is common to suffer visual variations while the eye adapts to its new lens. This might involve transient visual alterations like halos or glare around lights, which usually improve over time as the eye heals.

Overall, the visual recovery and adaption time after cataract surgery varies from person to person; nevertheless, with patience and good care, most patients see considerable improvements in their eyesight and quality of life.

Benefits Of Improved Vision Following Surgery

The advantages of enhanced eyesight after cataract surgery are many, and they may have a significant influence on a person's quality of life. Here are some of the main benefits:

1. Clearer eyesight: One of the most noticeable advantages of cataract surgery is improved eyesight. Many patients report major improvements in their ability to see items at varied distances, from reading to driving.

2. Improved Quality of Life: Many patients report that having sharper eyesight enhances their overall quality of life. They may be able to engage in activities that they previously loved but were unable to perform because of impaired eyesight.

3. Increased Independence: Improved eyesight may lead to more independence. Patients may no longer need help with everyday activities including reading, cooking, or navigating their environment.

4. Reduced Risk of Falls and Accidents: Poor eyesight may heighten the risk of falls and accidents, particularly in older persons. Cataract surgery may improve eyesight and minimize the likelihood of these events.

5. Improved Social Interaction: Having clearer eyesight makes it simpler to participate in social events and maintain connections with friends and family. Patients may feel more secure in social situations if they can see properly.

6. Better Mental Health: Poor eyesight may hurt mental health, causing feelings of frustration, loneliness, and sadness. By enhancing eyesight, cataract surgery may help reduce unpleasant feelings and enhance general mental health.

Overall, the advantages of better eyesight after cataract surgery go well beyond just seeing more clearly. It has the potential to improve a person's life, giving them more freedom, confidence, and overall pleasure.

Tips To Maintain Eye Health And Prevent Future Cataracts

While cataract surgery may enhance vision, it is essential to take precautions to preserve eye health and avoid more cataracts. Here are some helpful tips:

1. Protect Your Eyes from UV Rays: The sun's ultraviolet (UV) rays increase the risk of cataracts. Wear sunglasses that block 100% of UVA and UVB rays while you're outside, even on overcast days.

2. Quit smoking: Smoking is a significant risk factor for cataracts and other eye problems. If you smoke, stopping may help lower your chances of having cataracts in the future.

3. Consume a Healthy Diet: A diet rich in fruits and vegetables, especially those strong in antioxidants such as vitamins C and E, may help avoid cataracts. Include a variety of colored fruits and vegetables in your diet to promote eye health.

4. Maintain a Healthy Weight: Being overweight or obese raises the risk of cataracts. To maintain a healthy weight and lower your risk, eat a well-balanced diet and exercise regularly.

5. Manage Chronic Conditions: Diabetes and high blood pressure might raise the risk of cataracts. Work with your healthcare physician to successfully manage these disorders and reduce their influence on your eye health.

6. **Get Regular Eye examinations:** Regular eye examinations are critical for recognizing eye issues early on and tracking vision changes. Schedule regular eye examinations with an eye care specialist, even if you don't have any visual concerns.

By following these recommendations, you may help safeguard your eyes and lower your chances of acquiring cataracts in the future. Taking proactive efforts to preserve eye health is critical for maintaining eyesight and a great quality of life.

Resources For Ongoing Support And Education

Following cataract surgery, it is critical to have continued care and education to promote optimum eye health and recovery. Here are some resources that might be useful:

1. **Support Groups:** Joining a support group for those who have had cataract surgery may give significant

emotional support as well as practical advice for getting through life after surgery. These organizations may meet in person or online.

2. **Educational resources:** Many organizations, including eye care providers and non-profit groups, provide educational resources regarding cataracts, cataract surgery, and eye health. These materials might include brochures, booklets, and internet information.

3. **Follow-up Care:** After cataract surgery, make sure you attend all planned follow-up sessions with your eye care specialist. These sessions are critical for monitoring your eye health and ensuring that your rehabilitation is going as planned.

4. **Patient Advocacy Organizations:** The American Academy of Ophthalmology and Prevent Blindness provides information and assistance to those living with cataracts and other eye disorders. These organizations may provide information about

treatment alternatives, financial aid programs, and advocacy initiatives.

By using these tools, you may remain up to date on cataract surgery and eye health while also connecting with people who can give support and help along the road. Remember that you are not alone on your journey, and there are several tools available to assist you navigate life after cataract surgery.

Conclusion

In conclusion, understanding cataract surgery is critical for patients, caregivers, and healthcare providers. This complex treatment, although routine and typically safe, needs much expertise and awareness to provide the best results and patient satisfaction.

First and foremost, cataracts must be recognized as a cause of vision impairment. Cataracts are not an unavoidable result of aging, but rather a curable disorder that has a substantial influence on a person's quality of life. Understanding the signs and evolution of cataracts allows individuals to seek prompt treatment and enhance their visual function.

Second, the advancement of surgical methods and technology has transformed cataract therapy. From classic extra capsular extraction to advanced phacoemulsification, surgeons today have a wealth of alternatives for tailoring the treatment to each patient's unique circumstances. Furthermore, advances like femtosecond laser-assisted cataract surgery and premium intraocular lenses increase accuracy and visual results, hence increasing patient satisfaction.

Furthermore, informing patients about the surgical procedure and its dangers is critical for making educated decisions. Healthcare practitioners may reduce anxiety and establish confidence with patients having cataract surgery by encouraging open conversation and addressing their concerns. Furthermore, including caregivers in preoperative and postoperative care creates a supportive atmosphere for the patient's rehabilitation.

Furthermore, postoperative care and rehabilitation are critical to achieving optimal vision recovery and long-term results. Patients must follow drug regimens, attend follow-up visits, and make lifestyle changes to improve recovery and avoid problems. Healthcare practitioners may help their patients transition smoothly to better eyesight by stressing the significance of compliance and offering continuing assistance.

Finally, ongoing research and innovation are critical for developing the profession of cataract surgery. Researchers can improve the safety, effectiveness, and accessibility of cataract surgery for people all around the globe by conducting clinical studies, fine-tuning surgical procedures, and investigating innovative treatment options. Collaboration among multidisciplinary teams, which include ophthalmologists, researchers, engineers, and policymakers, is critical for advancing research and meeting the changing demands of cataract patients.

Comprehending cataract surgery involves more than simply the technical components of the technique. Comprehensive patient education, tailored treatment, and continual innovation are required to achieve the best possible results and quality of life for cataract patients. By adopting these concepts, we can continue to enhance the quality of treatment while also empowering patients to restore clarity and vision in their lives.

THE END

www.ingramcontent.com/pod-product-compliance
Lightning Source LLC
Chambersburg PA
CBHW071837210526
45479CB00001B/176